High Protein Bariatric Cookbook

Easy & Delicious Homemade Recipes for your Health

Peter Michtor

Table of Contents

Introduction

Welcome to the world of high protein bariatric cookery, a culinary adventure designed exclusively for people looking to adopt a healthy lifestyle following bariatric surgery. This cookbook is intended to be your go-to resource for delicious and nutritious dishes that support your specific dietary needs and weight loss goals.

Bariatric surgery is a life-changing treatment that can give those who are severely obese a new lease on life. The operation shrinks the stomach, allowing patients to feel fuller with fewer quantities and lose significant weight. It is critical to follow a post-surgery diet that not only supports healing but also increases nutrient intake while minimizing calorie consumption.

A high-protein diet is one of the pillars of a good post-bariatric lifestyle. Protein is the building block of life, supporting tissue repair, muscle upkeep, and a variety of other vital physiological activities. Protein is essential for bariatric patients to maintain lean muscle mass, enhance metabolism, and feel full while losing weight.

This cookbook has a delectable collection of recipes expertly developed by culinary specialists and healthcare professionals. These dishes create the ideal mix between delightful flavors and nutritious nutrients, guaranteeing that you never have to choose between pleasure and health.

Each recipe is deliberately created to fit within the constraints of your post-bariatric diet, from delectable breakfast options to filling lunch and dinner masterpieces. We've also included delectable snacks and sweets to ensure you have a variety of options for every occasion.

This cookbook also tries to address typical issues and obstacles encountered by bariatric patients during their gastronomic journey. We will teach you about portion control, necessary nutrient consumption, dietary consistency, and other practical ideas to help you get the most out of your bariatric lifestyle.

Remember, this cookbook isn't simply about calorie monitoring or following tight diets. It's about developing a new relationship with food that feeds both your body and your soul. We've selected recipes that are both delicious and nutritious, promoting the conviction that healthy eating can be both pleasant and sustainable.

So come along with us on this journey to rejuvenate your eating habits, discover new culinary delights, and enjoy the benefits of a high-protein bariatric diet. Let us go on a journey toward a better, happier, and more satisfying existence. Prepare to appreciate the sweetness one bite at a time.

Understanding the High Protein Bariatric Diet

A Guide to Weight Loss and Optimal Health

The high protein bariatric diet is a customized eating plan created for those who have had bariatric surgery, which is a life-changing technique used to treat severe obesity. This one-of-a-kind dietary approach is critical for post-surgery healing, weight management, and overall well-being. Bariatric patients can achieve long-term weight loss, muscle mass, and improved health by prioritizing protein intake while carefully controlling other nutrients.

Bariatric surgery modifies the digestive system by reducing stomach size to reduce food intake. Patients report reduced appetite and early satiety following the surgery, allowing them to consume lesser servings. This change, however, implies that their ability to absorb important nutrients, particularly proteins, may be compromised. As a result, the high protein bariatric diet appears as a strategic strategy to address their nutritional requirements while encouraging optimal weight loss outcomes.

Protein's Importance in the Bariatric Diet

Protein is the building block of tissue repair and maintenance, and it is essential for many body processes such as immunological support, enzyme manufacturing, and hormone regulation. Getting enough protein after bariatric surgery is critical for wound healing, preventing muscle loss, and providing the energy needed for daily activities.

Furthermore, protein has a distinct satiating impact, making people feel fuller for longer periods of time and decreasing the likelihood of overeating or taking too many calories. This is especially crucial for bariatric patients, whose lower stomach capacity necessitates nutrient-dense foods to meet their dietary needs.

Critical Elements of the High Protein Bariatric Diet

1. Lean Protein Sources: Bariatric patients are urged to eat lean protein sources such poultry, fish, lean cuts of meat, tofu, lentils, and low-fat dairy products. These solutions give plenty of protein without adding unwanted fats and calories.

2. Texture and Consistency: To aid in the healing process, patients initially take a diet consisting of soft and pureed meals. They can progressively reintroduce solid foods as time goes on, but it's critical to favor easily digestible items that won't tax the newly remodeled digestive system.

3. Nutrient Density: In a bariatric diet, every mouthful counts, and choosing nutrient-dense foods is critical to ensuring that patients satisfy their vitamin and mineral needs. To create a well-rounded and balanced diet, vegetables, fruits, and whole grains should be included alongside protein sources.

4. Portion management: Despite the physiological changes caused by surgery, portion management is still important. To avoid overstretching their stomach pouches and to maintain a consistent flow of nutrients throughout the day, bariatric patients must consume small, frequent meals.

5. Hydration: It's crucial to stay hydrated, but it's also important to avoid drinking with meals, which can wash food through the stomach too rapidly and cause discomfort.

The Advantages of a High Protein Bariatric Diet

The advantages of a high protein bariatric diet go far beyond weight loss. Patients frequently report increased energy, improved mood, improved physical mobility, and a lower risk of weight-related health issues such as diabetes, hypertension, and sleep apnea. Furthermore, by adopting this lifestyle, individuals can develop a good relationship with food, supporting a long-term dedication to their health and well-being.

To summarize, the high protein bariatric diet is a powerful tool that allows people to reclaim control of their health and life. Bariatric patients can embark on a journey to a better and more fulfilling future by concentrating on nutritional protein sources, mindful eating, and balanced nutrition. To personalize your dietary plan and achieve the best outcomes, always consult with healthcare specialists and nutritionists.

Remember that the key to success is to take one step at a time, to embrace progress, and to celebrate small successes along the road.

Tips and Strategies for Success in the High Protein Bariatric Diet

1. Consult a Registered Dietitian: Consult a qualified dietitian or nutritionist with experience in bariatric treatment before beginning the high protein bariatric diet. They can tailor your diet to your unique surgery, health situation, and individual requirements.

2. Make Protein-Rich Foods a Priority: Make lean protein the focal point of your meals. Include chicken, turkey, fish, eggs, low-fat dairy, tofu, and legumes as alternatives. These foods will keep you feeling fuller for longer and will help you maintain muscle mass.

3. Begin Texture Progression Slowly: Following surgery, your diet will most likely begin with liquids and progress to soft and pureed foods. To avoid discomfort, gradually reintroduce solid foods, taking your time to adjust to varied textures.

4. Spacing Meals throughout the Day: Eat small, frequent meals throughout the day to ensure a consistent supply of nutrients without overburdening your smaller stomach pouch.

5. Chew carefully and mindfully: To help digestion, chew each bite thoroughly. Eating consciously and without distractions allows you to realize when you're full and helps you avoid overeating.

6. Hydration Habits: Stay hydrated by sipping water throughout the day, but avoid drinking during meals to minimize stomach acid dilution and pouch stretching.

7. Investigate Protein Supplements: If you find it difficult to satisfy your protein needs through food alone, consult your dietician about protein supplements. Protein powders and shakes are examples of these.

8. Plan Balanced Meals: To make balanced and nutritious meals, combine lean proteins with vegetables, fruits, and whole grains.

9. Prepare Meals and Snacks: Prepare protein-rich meals and snacks ahead of time to make it simpler to keep to your diet plan, especially on hectic days.

10. Reduce Added Sugars and Fats: Reduce your intake of added sweets and bad fats, which can give empty calories and sabotage your weight loss efforts.

11. Experiment with different spices and herbs: To add flavor to your meals without adding calories, generously use spices and herbs. This keeps your taste buds stimulated and prevents meal boredom.

12. Remain Active: Regular physical activity helps to supplement the high protein bariatric diet and promotes greater weight loss and general health. Consult your healthcare team to choose the best exercises for your stage of recovery.

13. Keep Track of Nutrient Intake: Keep note of your food intake, particularly your vitamin and mineral intake.

Supplements may be required for bariatric patients to avoid deficiencies.

14. Stay Connected: Participate in support groups or online forums with other bariatric patients to exchange experiences, advice, and motivation as you progress through your journey.

15. Avoid Grazing and Snacking: Avoid grazing or snacking between meals, as this can result in unintentional calorie ingestion.

16. Practice Portion Control: Invest in smaller dishes and bowls to assist you efficiently regulate portion proportions.

17. Celebrate Non-Scale Victories: Recognize and celebrate accomplishments other than weight loss, such as greater energy, improved fitness, and overall well-being.

Keep in mind that the high protein bariatric diet is a long-term commitment to your health and weight loss.

Accept the process with patience and care to yourself, as development may be slow. When making big changes to your diet or lifestyle, always get advice from your healthcare team. You can succeed in your high protein bariatric journey and embark on a route to a healthier and more satisfying life with dedication, determination, and the appropriate tactics

High-Protein Bariatric Diet Dishes

Here are high-protein bariatric diet dishes with its ingredients and preparations:

Breakfast Burrito for Bariatric Patients:

Ingredients:
Scrambled eggs, turkey sausage, bell peppers, onions, and a whole wheat tortilla.

Preparations:
Fill a whole wheat tortilla with scrambled eggs, turkey sausage, sautéed bell peppers and onions, and serve. Roll it up and eat it.

Greek Yogurt Parfait:

Ingredients:
Greek yogurt, mixed berries, honey, and granola.

Preparations:

In a glass, layer Greek yogurt, mixed berries, and honey. For extra crunch, sprinkle with granola.

Protein-Rich Smoothie:

Ingredients:

Protein powder, almond milk, banana, spinach, and chia seeds.

Preparations:

Protein powder, almond milk, banana, spinach, and chia seeds should be blended until smooth.

Tuna Salad Lettuce Wraps:

Ingredients:

Canned tuna, Greek yogurt, celery, red onion, and lettuce leaves.

Preparations:

Combine canned tuna, Greek yogurt, celery, and red onion. Serve wrapped in lettuce leaves.

Stuffed Quinoa Bell Peppers:

Ingredients:

Quinoa, lean ground turkey, bell peppers, and chopped tomatoes.

Preparations:

Cook the quinoa and lean ground turkey. Fill halved bell peppers with the mixture and bake until cooked.

Baked Chicken Breast:

Ingredients:

Chicken breast, olive oil, herbs and spices.

Preparations:

Rub the chicken breast with olive oil, herbs, and spices before cooking. Bake until well done.

Shrimp Stir-Fry:

Ingredients:

Shrimp, mixed vegetables, and low-sodium soy sauce

Preparations:

In a pan, stir-fry shrimp and mixed vegetables with low-sodium soy sauce.

Cottage Cheese and Fruit Salad:

Ingredients:

Cottage cheese, assorted fruits (such as berries and melon).

Preparations:

To make a delicious snack, top cottage cheese with assorted fruits.

Turkey Meatballs:

Ingredients:

Ground turkey, egg, breadcrumbs, and Italian herbs.

Preparations:

Combine ground turkey, egg, breadcrumbs, and Italian herbs in a mixing bowl. Bake the meatballs after they have been formed.

Protein-Rich Omelette:

Ingredients:

Eggs, chopped ham, spinach, and low-fat cheese.

Preparations:

Prepare the eggs by whisking them and pouring them into a pan. Toss in the diced ham, spinach, and low-fat cheese. Cook until the mixture is set.

Baked Salmon:

Ingredients:

Salmon fillet, lemon, and dill.

Preparations:

Place the salmon fillet on a baking sheet, drizzle with lemon juice, and sprinkle with dill. Bake until well done.

Chickpea Salad:

Ingredients:

Chickpeas, cucumber, cherry tomatoes, feta cheese, olive oil, and lemon juice.

Preparations:

Combine chickpeas, cucumber, cherry tomatoes, and feta cheese in a mixing bowl. Drizzle with lemon juice and olive oil.

Protein-Packed Pancakes:

Ingredients:

Protein powder, egg, banana, and almond milk.
Blend the protein powder, egg, banana, and almond milk together. Cook like you would regular pancakes.

Stir-Fry of Tofu and Vegetables:

Ingredients:

Firm tofu, mixed vegetables, and teriyaki sauce.

Preparations:

In a pan, stir-fry firm tofu and mixed vegetables with teriyaki sauce.

Lettuce Wraps with Egg Salad:

Ingredients:

Hard-boiled eggs, Greek yogurt, mustard, and lettuce leaves.

Preparations:

Mash hard-boiled eggs with Greek yogurt and mustard to make a mash. Serve wrapped in lettuce leaves.

Grilled Chicken Skewers:

Ingredients:

Chicken breast, bell peppers, and red onion.

Preparations:

Thread the chicken breast, bell peppers, and red onion onto skewers and set aside. Grill until well cooked.

Salad with Black Beans and Quinoa:

Ingredients:

Black beans, quinoa, sliced bell peppers, lime juice, and cilantro.

Preparations:

To make a substantial salad, combine black beans, quinoa, diced bell peppers, lime juice, and cilantro.

Salad with Eggs and Avocado:

Ingredients:

Hard-boiled eggs, avocado, cherry tomatoes, and balsamic vinegar.

Preparations:

Chop the hard-boiled eggs, avocado, and cherry tomatoes. Mix in the balsamic vinegar.

Soup with Chicken and Vegetables:

Ingredients:

Chicken broth, shredded chicken, and mixed veggies.

Preparations:

To make a hearty soup, simmer chicken broth, shredded chicken, and mixed veggies.

Greek Chicken Pita:

Ingredients:

Grilled chicken, cucumber, tomato, feta cheese, whole wheat pita.

Preparations:

Fill a whole wheat pita with grilled chicken, cucumber, tomato, and feta cheese to make a sandwich.

Spinach and Feta Stuffed Chicken Breast:

Ingredients:

Chicken breast, spinach, and feta cheese.

Preparations:

Prepare the chicken breast by stuffing it with sautéed spinach and feta cheese. Bake until well done.

Lentil Soup:

Ingredients:

Lentils, carrots, celery, and vegetable broth.

Preparations:

To prepare a healthful soup, cook lentils with carrots, celery, and vegetable broth.

Turkey and Avocado Wrap:

Ingredients:

Turkey slices, avocado, lettuce leaves, and a whole wheat wrap.

Preparations:

Prepare a whole wheat wrap by layering turkey slices, avocado, and lettuce leaves. Roll it up and eat it.

Herbed Baked Cod:

Ingredients:

Cod fillet, garlic, thyme, and lemon.

Preparations:

Place the cod fillet on a baking sheet, season with garlic and thyme, and top with lemon slices. Bake until well done.

Salad with Mozzarella and Tomatoes:

Ingredients:

Fresh mozzarella, cherry tomatoes, basil leaves, and balsamic glaze.

Preparations:

Layer fresh mozzarella, cherry tomatoes, and basil leaves in a serving dish. Drizzle the balsamic glaze over the top.

Black Bean Burger with Protein:

Ingredients:

Black beans, egg, breadcrumbs, onions, and a whole wheat bun.

Preparations:

Mash black beans with an egg, breadcrumbs, and onions. Make patties and fry in a skillet. On a whole wheat bun, serve.

Herb-Baked Halibut:

Ingredients:

Halibut fillet, rosemary, oregano, and lemon.

Preparations:

Place the halibut fillet on a baking sheet, season with rosemary and oregano, and top with lemon slices. Bake until well done.

Casserole with Cheesy Cauliflower:

Ingredients:

Cauliflower florets, low-fat cheese, Greek yogurt, and garlic.

Preparations:

Combine cauliflower florets, low-fat cheese, Greek yogurt, and garlic in a mixing bowl. Bake until the potatoes are soft and cheesy.

Stuffed Mushrooms with Turkey and Spinach:

Ingredients:

Ground turkey, spinach, and mushrooms.

Preparations:

Fill mushroom caps with a mixture of cooked ground turkey and spinach. Bake until the potatoes are soft.

Spinach and Ricotta Stuffed Chicken Breast:

Ingredients:

Chicken breast, ricotta cheese, spinach.

Preparations:

Prepare the chicken breast by stuffing it with ricotta cheese and sautéed spinach. Bake until well done.

Baked Zucchini Boats with Ground Turkey:

Ingredients:

Zucchini, ground turkey, chopped tomatoes, and low-fat cheese.

Preparations:

Prepare the zucchini by hollowing it out and filling it with a mixture of cooked ground turkey and diced tomatoes. Bake until the zucchini is soft.

Serve with low-fat dressing.

Protein-Rich Overnight Oatmeal:

Ingredients:

Rolled oats, Greek yogurt, chia seeds, and almond milk.

Preparations:

In a jar, combine rolled oats, Greek yogurt, chia seeds, and almond milk. Refrigerate overnight, then serve in the morning.

Salad with Shrimp and Avocado:

Ingredients:

Shrimp, avocado, cherry tomatoes, cilantro, and lime juice.

Preparations:

To make a delicious salad, combine cooked shrimp, avocado, cherry tomatoes, cilantro, and lime juice.

Protein-Packed Chicken Salad:

Ingredients:

Shredded chicken, Greek yogurt, celery, grapes, and almonds.

Preparations:

To make a tasty chicken salad, combine shredded chicken, Greek yogurt, chopped celery, grapes, and almonds.

Lemon Garlic Grilled Shrimp:

Ingredients:

Shrimp, lemon juice, garlic, and olive oil.

Preparations:

Marinate the shrimp in lemon juice, garlic, and olive oil. Grill until well cooked.

Stir-Fry with Turkey and Vegetables:

Ingredients:

Ground turkey, mixed veggies, and soy sauce.

Preparations:

In a pan, stir-fry ground turkey and mixed vegetables with soy sauce.

Baked Tofu Nuggets:

Ingredients:

Firm tofu, whole wheat breadcrumbs, and paprika.

Preparations:

Coat firm tofu slices with whole wheat breadcrumbs and paprika before baking. Bake until the bacon is crispy.

Chicken Fajita Bowl:

Ingredients:

Grilled chicken, bell peppers, onions, quinoa, and salsa.

Preparations:

Cooked quinoa is topped with grilled chicken, sautéed bell peppers, onions, and salsa.

Tofu with Vegetable Skewers:

Ingredients:

Firm tofu, bell peppers, and zucchini.

Preparations:

Thread firm tofu, bell peppers, and zucchini onto skewers to prepare. Grill the tofu until it is gently browned.

High Protein Chocolate Pudding:

Ingredients:

Silken tofu, cocoa powder, honey, and vanilla essence.

Preparations:

To make the silken tofu, combine it with the chocolate powder, honey, and vanilla essence until smooth. Allow to cool before serving.

Grilled Steak with Asparagus:

Ingredients:

Sirloin steak, asparagus, olive oil, and garlic.

Preparations:

Season the meat with garlic and olive oil before cooking.

Grill the meat and asparagus until cooked through.

Tofu Scramble:

Ingredients:

Firm tofu, bell peppers, onions, and turmeric.

Preparations:

To make a nice scramble, crumble firm tofu and sauté with

bell peppers, onions, and turmeric.

Stuffed Portobello Mushrooms with Spinach and Feta:

Ingredients:

Portobello mushrooms, spinach, and feta cheese.

Preparations:

Stuff Portobello mushrooms with sautéed spinach and feta cheese before baking. Bake until the mushrooms are soft.

Protein-Packed Cheesy Broccoli Soup:

Ingredients:

Broccoli, low-fat cheese, chicken broth.

Preparations:

Cook broccoli in chicken stock, then combine with low-fat cheese to make a creamy soup.

Lettuce Wraps with Shrimp and Avocado:

Ingredients:

Shrimp, avocado, cucumber, and lettuce leaves.

Preparations:

Combine cooked shrimp, diced avocado, and cucumber in a mixing bowl. Serve wrapped in lettuce leaves.

Stuffed Bell Peppers with Ground Chicken:

Ingredients:

Ground chicken, quinoa, diced tomatoes, and bell peppers.

Preparations:

Combine cooked ground chicken, quinoa, and diced tomatoes in a mixing bowl. Bake the mixture stuffed into halved bell peppers.

Baked Almond Crusted Fish:

Ingredients:

White fish fillet, almond flour, and lemon zest.

Preparations:

Coat the fish fillet with almond flour and lemon zest before cooking. Bake until the fish is well done.

Black Bean and Chicken Lettuce Wraps:

Ingredients:

Shredded black beans, shredded chicken, lettuce wraps, and black beans, avocado, lettuce leaves.

Preparations:

Prepare by combining shredded chicken and black beans. Serve in lettuce leaves with avocado slices.

Turkey and Quinoa Stuffed Zucchini:

Ingredients:

Ground turkey, cooked quinoa, and zucchini.

Preparations:

Prepare the zucchini by hollowing it out and filling it with a mixture of cooked ground turkey and quinoa. Bake until the zucchini is soft.

High Protein Egg Salad Wrap:

Ingredients:

Hard-boiled eggs, Greek yogurt, mustard, and a whole wheat wrap.

Preparations:

Chop hard-boiled eggs and combine with Greek yogurt and mustard. Wrap in a whole wheat tortilla and serve.

Baked Chicken and Vegetable Casserole:

Ingredients:

Chicken breast, mixed veggies, and low-sodium chicken broth.

Preparations:

Arrange the chicken breast and mixed veggies in a baking dish. Bake until the chicken is cooked through, then pour over the low-sodium chicken broth.

Cauliflower Fried Rice with Shrimp:

Ingredients:

Cauliflower rice, shrimp, mixed vegetables, and soy sauce.

Preparations:

To make low-carb fried rice alternative, stir-fry shrimp, mixed vegetables, and cauliflower rice with soy sauce.

Salad with Tuna and White Beans:

Ingredients:

Canned tuna, white beans, cherry tomatoes, and red onion.

Preparations:

Combine canned tuna, white beans, cherry tomatoes, and red onion in a mixing bowl. Drizzle with lemon juice and olive oil.

Spinach and Feta Stuffed Turkey Meatloaf:

Ingredients:

Ground turkey, spinach, feta cheese, and diced tomatoes.

Preparations:

Combine ground turkey, cooked spinach, feta cheese, and diced tomatoes in a mixing bowl. Form into a loaf and bake until well done.

Stir-Fry of Lentils and Vegetables:

Ingredients:

Cooked lentils, mixed vegetables, and teriyaki sauce.

Preparations:

In a pan, stir-fry cooked lentils and mixed vegetables with teriyaki sauce.

Tofu & Veggie Lettuce Wraps:

Ingredients:

Firm tofu, julienned carrots, cucumber, and lettuce leaves.

Preparations:

Sauté firm tofu with julienned carrots and cucumber in a skillet. Serve wrapped in lettuce leaves.

Lemon Herb Butter Baked Cod:

Ingredients:

Cod fillet, butter, lemon juice, herbs (e.g., parsley, thyme).

Preparations:

Arrange the cod fillets on a baking sheet. Melted butter, lemon juice, and herbs should be combined. Brush the fish with the sauce and bake until done.

High Protein Berry Chia Pudding:

Ingredients:

Greek yogurt, chia seeds, and mixed berries.

Preparations:

Prepare by combining Greek yogurt with chia seeds. Refrigerate until the berries have reached a pudding-like consistency.

Stir-Fried Chicken with Broccoli:

Ingredients:

Chicken breast, broccoli, and low-sodium soy sauce.

Preparations:

Cook the chicken breast and broccoli in a pan with low-sodium soy sauce.

Salad with Zesty Shrimp and Avocado:

Ingredients:

Shrimp, avocado, cherry tomatoes, cilantro, lime juice, and jalapeo (optional).

Preparations:

To make a tasty salad, combine cooked shrimp, chopped avocado, cherry tomatoes, cilantro, lime juice, and jalapeo (if using).

These high protein bariatric diet dishes include a variety of flavors and ingredients to keep your meals interesting and filling. Always follow the advice of your healthcare provider and adjust these recipes to your specific nutritional needs and tastes. Take pleasure in your gastronomic path to better health and well-being.

Here's a 30-day meal plan using dishes from the list above:

Day 1:

- Breakfast: Breakfast for Bariatric Patients Burrito

- Greek Yogurt Parfait for Lunch

- Grilled Chicken Skewers with Asparagus for Dinner

Day 2:

- Smoothie with Protein for Breakfast

- Tuna Salad Lettuce Wraps for Lunch

- Quinoa Stuffed Bell Peppers for Dinner

Day 3:

- Cottage Cheese and Fruit Bowl for Breakfast

- Turkey Meatballs for Lunch

- Baked Salmon with Herbs for Dinner

Day 4:

- Protein-Packed Omelette for Breakfast

- Chickpea Salad for Lunch

- Spinach and Feta Stuffed Chicken Breast for Dinner

Day 5:

- Baked Chicken Breast for Breakfast

- Egg Salad Lettuce Wraps for Lunch

- Lentil Soup for Dinner

Day 6:

- Grilled Steak with Asparagus for Breakfast

- Protein-Packed Cheesy Broccoli Soup for Lunch

- Shrimp and Avocado Salad for Dinner

Day 7:

- Tofu Scramble for Breakfast

- Stuffed Bell Peppers with Ground Chicken for Lunch

- Almond Crusted Baked Fish for Dinner

Day 8:

- Black Bean and Chicken Lettuce Wraps for Breakfast

- Lunch: Stuffed Zucchini with Turkey and Quinoa

- Baked Chicken and Vegetable Casserole for Dinner

Day 9:

- High Protein Egg Salad for Breakfast

Lunch Wrap: Cauliflower Fried Rice with Shrimp

- Tuna and White Bean Salad for Dinner

Day 10:

- Breakfast: Stuffed Portobello Mushrooms with Spinach and Feta

- Spinach and Ricotta Stuffed Chicken Breast for Lunch

- Baked Cod with Lemon Herb Butter for Dinner

Day 11:

- Protein-Rich Pancakes for Breakfast

- Lentil and Vegetable Stir-Fry for Lunch

- For dinner, make a cheesy cauliflower casserole.

Day 12:

- Tofu and Veggie Lettuce Wraps for Breakfast

- Baked Tofu Nuggets for Lunch

- Pita with grilled chicken for dinner

Day 13:

- Protein-Packed Black Bean Burger for Breakfast

- Baked Halibut with Herbs for Lunch

- Turkey and Avocado Wrap for Dinner

Day 14:

- High Protein Chocolate Pudding for Breakfast

- Greek Chicken Pita for Lunch

- Protein for dinner-Overnight Oatmeal

Day 15:

- Shrimp Stir-Fry for Breakfast

- Egg and Avocado Salad for Lunch

- Salad with Mozzarella and Tomatoes for Dinner

Day 16:

- Breakfast: Breakfast Burrito for Bariatric Patients

- Greek Yogurt Parfait for Lunch

- Grilled Chicken Skewers with Asparagus for Dinner

Day 17:

- Smoothie with Protein for Breakfast

- Tuna Salad Lettuce Wraps for Lunch

- Quinoa Stuffed Bell Peppers for Dinner

Day 18:

- Cottage Cheese and Fruit Bowl for Breakfast

- Turkey Meatballs for Lunch

- Baked Salmon with Herbs for Dinner

Day 19:

- Protein-Packed Omelette for Breakfast

- Chickpea Salad for Lunch

- Spinach and Feta Stuffed Chicken Breast for Dinner

Day 20:

- Baked Chicken Breast for Breakfast

- Egg Salad Lettuce Wraps for Lunch

- Lentil Soup for Dinner

For the remaining days of your 30-day meal plan, rotate these delicious and nutritious high protein bariatric diet dishes.

Remember to alter the portion amounts and ingredients to your unique nutritional needs and goals. Take pleasure in your road to a better you.

Conclusion

Congratulations on finishing this delectable 30-day high protein bariatric diet meal plan! You have definitely experienced the power of healthful and tasty meals that fuel both your body and soul as you reflect on your culinary adventure. The mix of nutritional protein sources and carefully selected components has not only helped you achieve your weight loss objectives, but it has also improved your general well-being.

You've seen the transformative power of the high protein bariatric diet throughout this trip. You've empowered yourself to overcome problems and embark on a path to a better, happier life by prioritizing lean protein, vivid vegetables, and nutrient-dense foods. Each recipe has demonstrated that eating healthily does not have to mean sacrificing flavor, and that sustainable dietary choices can be both pleasurable and gratifying.

Remember the essential principles that have guided you along this route as you continue your post-bariatric lifestyle: portion control, careful eating, and staying hydrated. These simple yet effective tactics have assisted you in developing a positive relationship with food, ensuring that your meals nourish both your body and your spirit.

Your trip does not come to an end here. With your newfound knowledge and culinary creativity, you can continue to explore the world of high protein bariatric cuisine's limitless possibilities. The possibilities are endless, whether you're experimenting with new ingredients, tailoring recipes to your preferences, or discovering novel methods to combine nutrition and flavor.

Accept this closure as a new beginning, a new chapter in your life in which you honor your commitment to yourself and your health. Celebrate every accomplishment, no matter how minor, since it represents progress toward being the best version of yourself.

Remember that health is a continual and dynamic process as you move forward. It's about enjoying the journey, remaining strong in the face of disappointments, and cherishing the sense of accomplishment that comes with each step toward your goals.

You are not alone on this journey. The encouragement and motivation provided by fellow bariatric patients, healthcare experts, and loved ones will be priceless.

So, walk into this new chapter with fresh zeal, knowing that you have the skills to nourish your body and nurture your soul. You're not just sustaining your physical body when you relish each delectable bite; you're also embracing a lifestyle that fosters growth, resilience, and a profound appreciation for the gift of well-being.

May this conclusion represent the start of a thriving journey towards a healthy you, a journey filled with nutritious foods, bright tastes, and limitless possibilities. Trust in your inner strength and allow it to lead you to a life of sustenance, joy, and contentment. Accept the splendor of this chapter and the many chapters yet to unfold. Your path to optimal health and happiness has just begun, and it holds

the promise of endless moments to savor, one nourishing
step at a time.